Cure Adrenal Fatigue Now!

How to Diagnose & Overcome This Modern Day Stress Syndrome

By Dr Alex Nelson

Disclaimer

This book is intended to be a general guide, to raise
awareness, and to help people make informed decisions in
the context of their own personal circumstance. As
everybody's circumstances are different, so are the remedies
you should seek. While many of the recommendations in this
book can be applied by almost anybody regardless of their
conditions they are not intended to and should not be relied
upon to replace personal medical advice.
The author accepts no responsibility for any loss or injury, be
it personal or financial, as a result for the use or misuse of
the information in this book. If you have any doubts or
concerns after reading this book, please speak to a doctor or
other qualified person before taking any actions.

From The Author

Thank you for taking the time to read this book. As an
author, I understand the importance of creating books which
my readers will find both enjoyable and informative. If you
have the time and feel generous, please don't hesitate to
leave an honest review of this book.........Dr Alex Nelson.

Contents

Introduction

Chapter 1
What Is Adrenal Fatigue?

Chapter 2
The Symptoms Of Adrenal Fatigue

Chapter 3
What Are The Of Causes Adrenal Fatigue?

Chapter 4
Who Is Most Susceptible To Adrenal Fatigue?

Chapter 5
How To Determine If You Have Adrenal Fatigue

Chapter 6
The Effects Of Lifestyle & Nutrition On Adrenal Fatigue

Introduction

Have you ever heard about adrenaline rush or should I say do you enjoy adrenaline rushes and get bored when you don't have any crisis to handle? Are you struggling from anxiety, depression or in despair? Do you sometimes feel sleepy and tired without any pertinent reason?

If I could imagine a picture of you, it would be a haggard, disheveled, unkempt and emaciated. It may look like you own all the problems in the world. Oh my! The odds are you may have what people say: Adrenal Fatigue. A disorder identified by traditional medicine, eastern medicine and other alternative dynamic curative approach that briefly perceives this as a contemporary stress condition.

According to a source, 80% of American society today is confronting adrenal fatigue at a certain degree in their lives. Up until now, we were still unfamiliar of this dilemma. They merely assume that they don't feel good or think there are possible manifestations that draw them to investigate a diverse chaos. We always conclude that frequent symptoms designate various potential causes and every now and then (not sure what you are trying to say here, but imbricate is probably not the word) our affliction. Your daily choices and decisions in life can either abuse or alter the balance of your precious adrenal glands. If this part of your body get's too maltreated, that leads to Adrenal Fatigue.

Chapter 1
What Is Adrenal Fatigue?

Adrenal fatigue is also known as hypoadrenia or adrenal exhaustion: common terms used in traditional medicine. In the medical field, they refer to it as adrenal apathy, adrenal neurasthenia, neurasthenia, subclinical hypoadrenia or non-addison's hypoadrenia. Although this ailment already disturbs millions of people around the world, medical society doesn't acknowledge adrenal fatigue as a specific problem.

Adrenal fatigue is referred to as an accumulation and a mix of the colossal signs and symptoms which emerge from an alteration of the function of the adrenaline glands and a condition broadly attributed as a syndrome. This happens when you welcome anything that causes stress which can dominate and captivate your existence. In addition, Adrenal Fatigue is also a term used to give a reason for categorizing symptoms that are uttered by people who belong to the continuing stress of our well being. Some say you may be more prone to acquire this health issue if you are stressed with your job, a working student, single parent, a shift worker, or have squandered in alcohol and drugs.

As the term implies, the predominant sign of the ailment is fatigue. Different from the typical fatigue we experience this cannot be dealt with, by merely sleeping. Furthermore, you cannot immediately distinguish this as with other common diseases such as rubella. The feeling of exasperation will unrelentingly allure you down proceeding to quiescence of functional endeavor such as work.

Chapter 2
What Are The Symptoms of Adrenal Fatigue?

Too much physical, emotional, environmental and/or psychological stress can hurt your adrenals, causing a decrease in the output of adrenal hormones, especially cortisol.

> ➤ The primary symptom of adrenal fatigue is sustained fatigue that is not alleviated by sufficient amplitude of sleep or rest.

> ➤ Feeling of weakness or extreme fatigue and weary for no discernible rationale on a routine basis.

> ➤ Having difficulty getting out of bed in the morning, even when you had a reasonable amount of sleep.

- Morning fatigue – a person without a doubt intends to "wake up" as late as 10 a.m., but is indeed awake since 7 a.m.

- Afternoon "low" fatigue – apprehension of sleepiness or clouded thinking from 2 to 4 p.m.
  "Brain Fogs" the usage of the word "fogs" means you are literally imagining it. It is as if the cloud is making its way down through your thoughts making you less capable of thinking with clarity. A condition wherein there is absence of focus, being close, but it seems to be distant which causes an individual to extremely and consistently have the inability to remember and mental

disorientation where an individual is unable to have intellectual lucidity.

- Blast of energy at 6 p.m. -- You are finally excelling better from your afternoon activities.

- Sleepiness at 9 to 10 p.m. -- However, you can withstand going to sleep.

- "Second wind" that comes at around 11 p.m. which lasts just before 1 a.m., when you finally go to sleep. ***You have more energy and feel more alert in the evening. However, this is true only in the early stages of adrenal fatigue. If you have advanced to the more severe stage of adrenal exhaustion, you don't have energy at any point of the day, including the evening. Inability to handle stress is another classic hallmark in the list of adrenal fatigue symptoms.

  ➤ Slow to recuperate from an illness or stressful situations.

  ➤ Extreme hankering or a strong desire for salty food or sweets.

  ➤ Inability to lose weight or weight gain, particularly around the waist area.

  ➤ Lightheadedness (also known postural hypotension or orthostatic hypotension) when you suddenly stand up or stretch from a sitting position.

➤The requirement for stimulants to perform effectively in the morning and manage oneself all throughout the day.

➤Trembling when stressed out.

➤Increase in PMS (pre-menstrual syndrome) symptoms of menstrual flow that occurs consistently during the ten days prior to menses and vanishes either shortly before or shortly after the start of menstrual flow.

➤Feeling of convalescence momentarily after eating.

➤Frequent manifestations of flu or other respiratory conditions such as asthma and etc.

➤Memory loss and forgetfulness at all times.

➤Sense of being too tired to savor life.

Other symptoms of adrenal fatigue may include:

➤Feeling better when not dealing with stress
➤Back or neck pain with no probable reason
➤Difficulty in achieving daily tasks
➤Food allergies
➤Low sex drive
➤Dry skin
➤Nervousness
➤Constipation and/or diarrhea
➤Heart Palpitations
➤Mild Depression

➢Anxiety
➢Hair Loss
➢Low blood sugar level (hypoglycemia)
➢Loss of stamina and muscle strength

There are also conditions that are correlated with adrenal fatigue. If the adrenal glands become weak and impaired, the primary determinant in the medical and psychiatric disorders includes:

➢**Mental exhaustion-**The inability of the adrenal glands to function normally due to the intense and frequent nerve-racking circumstances faced by an individual in daily life.

➢**Multiple chemistry sensitivity-**This basically means that it is an acquired disorder that the burgeoning numbers of people including myself as well are having early onsets of health issues due to wide exposures of chemicals we are commonly using in our everyday life. So, once a person is exposed to it he/she may have recurring symptoms attributed to different organs in our body that are developing from reactions evident from being exposed to chemicals in a quantity that is significantly above the approved measurement for the general population. Enzyme and liver detoxification pathways may become overburdened affecting our system.

Once reactions are foreseen, occurrence of depression, fatigue, headache, migraines, difficulty concentrating, irritability, short term memory loss, lack of

6

coordination, shaking, trembling, visual and verbal disturbances, muscle pain, difficulty breathing, rashes, anxiety, impaired mobility, itching, disorientation, confusion, food sensitivity, excessive drowsiness, constipation, diarrhea, earaches, heart pounding, hypothyroidism, learning disabilities, elevated blood pressure, increased pulse and many more will start to appear.

These chemicals can be found in scented laundry soap or fabric softener, treated fabric, perfume, cologne, disinfectants, pesticides, herbicides household cleansers, cigarette smoke, car exhaust, gas heat or other petroleum products, air fresheners, bleach, shampoos, toothpaste, food supply, new carpet, cosmetics and others.

➤**Chronic fatigue syndrome**-a psychological condition misunderstood by most medical practitioners and even those who are exposed to it. It is characterized as the perception that there are weights attached to the arms and legs which make a person essentially feel that any activity is an overwhelming task. There is absolute tiredness. This may vary from one individual to the other.

➤**Fibromyalgia syndrome**-conditions centered in the muscles, ligament and tendons, wherein if you ask a patient with where the specific location hurts, the conventional answer would be "everywhere". Medical professionals had a lack of understanding and feel unequal to conclude and classify this condition as a psychological problem instead of gathering sufficient data and examining the legitimate authenticity of the problem.

➢**Rheumatoid Arthritis** – chronic inflammation that mainly affects the small joints in your hands and feet.

➢**Generalized anxiety disorders** – neurological disorders that are described to be the uncontrolled and often irrational worry.

➢**Hormonal imbalances** – occurring often times between 30s and 40s of both women and men. This may occur in teenagers once exposed to high levels of toxins and hormones that interrupt the normal action in the endocrine system. Hormones play a major role in regulating thought processes, mood, metabolism, growth, prenatal development, sexual development and function, metabolism, tissue function and psychological problems such depression, anxiety, memory and other mood related disorders.

➢**Deficiency in neurotransmitters** – the neurotransmitters serves as a line of connection to and from the body, mind and the central nervous system.

➢**Hypothyroidism** - The thyroid and the adrenal glands are co-dependent with one another. The normal function of the thyroid gland is reliant to how well the adrenal glands are working. Health practitioners should first take into consideration assessing their adrenal glands because it absolutely lowers the thyroid hormones once the adrenal glands are fragile or weak.

In addition, trying to push through with a thyroid treatment when the adrenal glands cannot carry out its function can cause the adrenal glands to collapse and result in the worsening condition in health. Once an individual starts taking in synthetic thyroid hormones and experiencing side effects, the problem is more likely to be found in the adrenal glands.

➢**Hypoglycemia** – when the adrenal glands cannot function normally and won't be able to convert glycogen to sugar properly once the insulin has been released, the adrenal glands then have to send the neurotransmitters to inform the pancreas to stop secreting insulin. When the adrenal glands are exhausted, they become slow or late in functioning which permits the overproduction of insulin resulting in blood sugar levels that are too low.

➢**Candida overgrowth** – too weak adrenal glands can harbour Candida yeast to increase quickly in the body. Forcing and nonstop stress can make the adrenal glands weak and continuing to affect the immune system.

➢Depression that may be situational and biochemical.

➢Allergies

➢Frequent infections

➢**Auto immune disorders** – abnormal immune responses from substances and tissues that are present in the body.

Chapter 3
What Are The Causes Of Adrenal Fatigue?

The cause of adrenal fatigue is not naturally simplified to one exact symptom, but is generally a combination of more than one of the following:

•Stress. Big adjustments in your life, a cumbersome workload that exceeds capabilities resulting in stress and also shabby diet practices.

•Not enough sleep. We usually find that our most restful sleep comes between 6-9am, right around the time we have to get up and ready for work or send kids off to school. Eventually, we force ourselves to mount up, which in turn stresses our adrenals and causes our first stress-induced cortisol release of the morning.

Cortisol is one of our stress-response hormones. Lack of sleep, or lack of good-quality sleep, influences the delivery of cortisol into our system. But, not in the way you probably think. We assume that if our glands were tired, their production levels decrease. However, sleep deprivation causes your body to release too much cortisol, for longer periods of time.

•Usually, the body has a cycle of release. The topmost levels in the morning which decline by the time you reach the evening. Your body may shoot up extra cortisol throughout the day if it recognizes physical and emotional stressors, but too much cortisol in the evening keeps you from experiencing periods of REM sleep causing you to wake up time and again overnight and wake up in the morning depleted of strength and energy.

Environmental toxins:

> ➤These include commonly used chemicals that are usually found in your personal care products, household cleaning supplies, plastic bottles, perfume, air fresheners, cologne, dishwashing soap, cosmetics, housing construction, laundry soap, pesticides, herbicides, etc. that contain endocrine disruptors (interferes with the body's endocrine system and produce adverse developmental, reproductive, neurological, and immune effects in both humans and wildlife) and are also a leading cause of adrenal fatigue.

> ➤Endocrine disruptors enter the body through our food, air and water attaching itself to our hormone receptor sites to impede normal functioning of the endocrine system. This, in turn, results in a variety of abnormal reactions throughout the body.
> **Note:** keeping the endocrine system in balance is a very delicate process and takes very little amount of toxins to cause damage.

> ➤In a few circumstances the disruptors tend to resemble hormones, which lead to overabundance. While in other cases, it serves as a barrier of hormones created or performing their responsibility in our system.

➤Our body is unable to break down these substances once they are ingested, inhaled, or entered our body. It is exceedingly very difficult and futile to eradicate. They compile in our tissues and adipose cells that constantly circle throughout our whole system.

➤Heavy metals, specifically mercury, instantly impede the production of the adrenal hormones.

•**Too little cholesterol and/or saturated fat in your diet and excessive carbohydrate intake:**

Our body was not designed to inherently ingest processed sugar, flour, junk foods, oil and other consumption goods because they have a negative nutritional content. If a person devours a diet deficient from the required nutrients needed by the body, this puts a constant burden on the adrenal glands together with the liver, pancreas and other organs.

If an individual eats refined products, it is rapidly absorbed by the body and contributes to the extreme increase of blood glucose levels. This fires an immediate signal to the pancreas to release excessive amount of insulin to compromise the uncontrolled high levels of blood sugar and gradually decrease blood sugar levels. Once this happens, the body then calls for the adrenal glands to release cortisol and bring the sugar levels back up because they work in tandem with the insulin to keep the blood sugar in balance. Anytime you indulge in eating sugar and refined foods the adrenals and the pancreas go through the same course and force excessive physiological demand onto them.

If the adrenal glands are summoned repeatedly to manage this dangerous sequence, the adrenal glands weaken and may not be able to release the adequate amount which is essential for functionality. In this matter, the blood sugar level is maintained in a consistent low level, but when fatigue and stress occur, this leads to the dilemma in hypoglycaemia.

●**Excessive caffeine or stimulant use:**
Caffeine usually heightens our stress hormones that prompt the production of nor epinephrine and epinephrine also known as the "fight or flight" response. In threatening or near fatal situations, these hormones yield us with the additional strength that we need, efficiency in stamina and vigilant to deal productively in situations impending. After a couple of hours from the ingestion of caffeine, the stress hormones are scattered in various directions and you may feel hungry, tired, ill-tempered and wanting more to grasp and indulge in caffeine. This will, in turn, make the exaggerated wear and tear of the adrenal glands over time cause fatigue.

On the other hand, Nicotine provokes the liver to produce an eminent amount of sugar. Increase in glucose level in the blood warns the pancreas release insulin to bring the sugar readings down. This results in the declining of blood sugar level and the excessive release of insulin and cortisol eventually burns-out the adrenal glands.

•Zinc deficiency:

When too many stresses occur, the adrenals can begin to breakdown. A lot of unfavorable consequences can stem from adrenal fatigue, including suppression of the immune function.

Zinc opposes the negative effects of stress and boost energy. When zinc is at a low level the adrenal glands are agitated, copper then is elevated and plays a role in adrenal problems. In this regard, during DNA synthesis and insulin production, zinc plays an important role as it impacts the adrenal glands, but up until now this was not scientifically proven.

•Sodium deficiency:

Once the symptoms are noticeable and are consistent, aside from cortisol and other stress hormones; other adrenal hormones such as sodium-sparring aldosterone may also fall.

The production of aldosterone instructs the kidneys to retain sodium in the bloodstream, which usually drops in such individuals. If unable to produce an ongoing supply of salt, their blood pressure may fall, resulting in dizziness when standing (postural hypotension) but, take note that the low-sodium state existing in adrenal fatigue does not account for all of the symptoms of adrenal fatigue, as fluctuations in cortisol also play a role.

Sodium is an essential nutrient to the function of the adrenal glands because the body cannot produce it. It helps in the sustenance of hydration and a steady blood pressure. Deficiency of sodium remains a rare condition because there is a wide supply of sodium by the form of tablets available in the pharmacy, commonly referred to as Sodium Chloride. Although many practitioners encourage less consumption of salt since it is a contributory to a lot of disorders. Active individuals lose an abundant amount of sodium when they sweat and thus require more sodium.

•A congenital weak adrenals:

Many children are born with this impairment because of the mothers' nutritional deficiencies since nutrients are passed through the placenta down to the unborn offspring. This is not a genetic problem. For instance, zinc deficiencies that are a common problem in mothers show that newborns have low zinc and often times are high in minerals such as copper, cadmium or substitute of zinc as well. By age 3 or 4, children may start to feel fatigue. They may get sick, depressed and most often have difficulty coping up in school. Some kids may react to a stimulus by becoming obsessive, hyperactive, compulsive hyperactive and developing behavioural problems. By testing mineral analysis through a strand of hair helps state whether or not they are burnout at this age, a new rare occurrence I would say. Refurbishing their body chemistry will generally vanish in a few months or years.

Chapter 4
Who is most susceptible to adrenal fatigue?

Anyone can have this ordeal in their lives. Debilitating diseases, crisis, ongoing endurance of difficult situations and depression can exhaust the adrenal glands reserves of even the healthiest person. Still, there are circumstances that can occur which will make you too receptive to adrenal fatigue. People that are in a dull status where they feel cornered or forlorn in their jobs, often in financial need, bad relationships, imprisonment for years and maternal fatigue during gestation either post term or mid-term pregnancy depression.

This may also be in individuals who have specific habits and lifestyles which include a very poor diet. Because each nutrient has a specific task to function in metabolism, dietary consumption patterns, requirement levels, and toxicity. Another is substance abuse, as with nicotine, alcohol, chemicals and drugs. Adrenal fatigue can also be seen in people who have little time to sleep and rest at least 8 hrs a day and, too many pressures which cause people to become unstable.

It may occur in people with coughs/colds that linger for several weeks and recurring bronchitis, pneumonia or other respiratory infections, asthma, colds, and other respiratory involvements two or more times per year. Women that have increasing symptoms of premenstrual syndrome (PMS) such as cramps, bloating, moodiness, irritability, emotional instability, headaches, tiredness, and/or intolerance before their period. Also, people who have dermatitis or other skin conditions, rheumatoid arthritis, people who have allergies to several things in the environment and multiple chemical sensitivities are susceptible to adrenal fatigue.

Stress will continue if we don't change our mindset to a positive outlook in life.

Chapter 5
How To Determine If You Have Adrenal Fatigue?

More often than not, blood chemistry or salivary testing is an option medical practitioners use to diagnose adrenal fatigue, but keep in mind that these tests are not backed with science since adrenal fatigue is not recognized as a medical condition.

Nearly all medical practitioners (including endocrinologists) are not efficient in determining if an individual has adrenal fatigue because they have their own framework on how they diagnose, treat and manage diseases they find. This is all based in theory. They have studied for many years, trained in prestigious universities or hospitals but they all base their findings on credible data and results from blood exams and procedures linking the symptoms verbalized by a patient with adrenal fatigue.

There is a blog post I read that states this:

"My doctor showed me a great little trick to test for adrenal fatigue. Take your blood pressure while sitting down and record the numbers. Keep the cuff around your arm and stand up. Take your blood pressure again immediately after standing. In a healthy person, the blood pressure will rise when they stand. In a person with adrenal fatigue, the blood pressure will drop when they stand."

Do you think that's true?

The most common and reliable method used for testing adrenal fatigue is "the saliva test". By the word itself, it is a method using the saliva of an individual. A kit can be directly ordered from the lab or a dispensing doctor can provide you with it and you can do it at home. You have to collect 4 different saliva samples and place them in a small vial or sample collection container. Saliva is collected around 7 am, 11 am, 4pm, and 11 pm. Once the specimens are complete send it to the laboratory for analysis and results may be claimed or mailed in your home. It is taken 4 times because the cortisol level fluctuates during the course of a day, and taking 4 samples will help you and your doctor to see if cortisol is increasing and dropping at the correct time frames.

Results from a saliva test is more preferable than a blood test to measure cortisol levels because through saliva, the active forms of hormones called the "free hormones" are measured whereas in blood tests, both inactive and active forms are measured looks like you have ample of hormones even though some are nonexistent in your body. But for adrenal fatigue, you may just want to look on the active and not the inactive adrenal hormones.

Be reminded as well that the adrenal glands and the thyroid glands work together, so this is hard to evaluate the results alone. A best approach to this is by identifying the most typical symptom and treats it until it diminishes. The results have a wide range and you may differ from somebody else, but are still considered normal. If you were told that you are at the low range from the normal level, there is still time for improvement. You might be testing if you are feeling better but when results come in, it may not be normal for you. If you have been in the high range for so long and suddenly drop down to normal when you feel good, it doesn't matter if your result has dropped by 25% or 50% but gauges in the normal range then that's normal for you.

Chapter 6
The Effects Of Lifestyle And Nutrition On Adrenal Fatigue

Stage	Response	Reaction
1) Alarm	•The adrenal glands always get notified when they sense stressors and their primary function is to secrete cortisol. •The Pancreas cells (insulin) are also altered reacting from inconsistent blood sugar levels. •The body is then rewarded in from heightened requirement for glucose.	Intense desire for foods rich in carbohydrates and fat. For example donuts, junk foods, carbonated drinks that has a very high glucose content, burgers and etc. Inability to sleep soundly and irritability begins to occur. This causes digestion of external substances that invigorates such as caffeine, alcohol, nicotine and refined foods. Other stimulants which include stress, environmental toxins (such as personal care products, cleaning supplies, perfume, air fresheners, cologne, dish soap, cosmetics, housing construction, laundry soap, pesticides, herbicides, etc. contain endocrine disruptors) and Candida overgrowth

2)Resistance	•If stressors prevail, the adrenal glands begin to feel overworked. This time it greatly hard to respond to the demand of cortisol in the body •Also, the thyroid glands start to act inappropriately. •In females, their ovaries begins to be impaired	Difficulty falling asleep and irritability when confronted with stress. Metabolism is impeded Sluggishness and weight gain begins to appear. PMS and menstrual irregularities in women. Mood swings for men.
3)Exhau-stion	•The adrenal gland starts to give up as it concedes to pressure. Cortisol levels start to decrease in production. •Body is in critical need for energy going further to breaking down its own muscles for protein	The body's aim is to survive by rapidly depleting resources. Fluctuation in blood pressure, digestion slows down and sexual drive begins to abate.

Chapter 7
How Traditional Medicine Approaches Adrenal Fatigue?

The key to successful treating of adrenal fatigue is an approach to use only gentle natural compounds along with dietary and lifestyle adjustments under proper professional supervision because improper usage of herbal supplements can also harm or alleviate the existing condition. Outcomes from traditional management will guide us. The body speaks to us, one way or another, we ourselves know if there is relief or not.

Why herbs?
This is because herbal compounds are older than human civilization. Animals consciously consume plants to compromise bacteria, viruses, parasites or worms. Humans too have a history that we are ingesting plants to support health and hunger.

Two ways to think about herbal treatment for adrenal fatigue:
a. Herbs can be used to modulate adrenal secretion (i.e., a "tonic" approach)
b. To increase the body's ability to respond to stress (an "adaptogenic" approach).

What follows are the most common and clinically effective herbs used in the treatment of adrenal fatigue.

Herbs excellent for maintaining homeostasis:

1.Rhodiola (Rhodiola rosea)

Rhodiola exerts these beneficial effects by regulating key mediators of the stress response including cortisol. This is an herb with a long history of traditional use. It acts in areas of stress and fatigue management, enhancement of mental performance and treatment of mild depression.

2.Korean ginseng (panax ginseng)

The main root is used in western herbal medicine to treat physical and mental exhaustion, assist in the adaptation of stress, improvement of insulin sensitivity, better memory, insomnia and fatigue in women with menopausal symptoms.

The recommended dose is 100mg, 1-4 times daily.
Note: insomnia – no panax ginseng later than midday

Without sleep problems: morning and early evening are well tolerated.

3.Ashwaganda (withania somnifera)

Useful for stress induced sleeping problems.
Note: high dose – 2g twice a day (take immediately prior bedtime)

Others:

1. **Licorice (Glycyrrhiza glabra and G. uralensis)**
   A friend to the adrenal cortex, a staple of traditional medicine for adrenal insufficiency and ulcers, this herb contains triterpenoid saponins that influence cortisol-cortisone balance throughout the body. Glycyrrhizin is the main active compound in licorice. At higher amounts, however, it has a strong effect on the kidney and allows cortisol to interact with aldosterone receptors, which affects sodium/potassium balance and increases blood pressure. For this reason, patients taking higher amounts of licorice need to be monitored closely.
   Note: 1.75 – 5.25 g per day = 25-75 mg per day

2. **Ginkgo (Ginkgo biloba)**
   Often overlooked is the fact that Ginkgo can favorably affect stress levels, it lowered cortisol levels in healthy patients undergoing glucose tolerance testing.
   Note: dose: 120 - 240 mg per day, given in divided doses (i.e. morning and evening, either with or without food.)

3. **Eleuthero (eleutherococcus senticosus)**
   Used for supporting cognition, alertness, physical stress and the ability to increase levels of stress protective heat shock proteins or the mild stressors of the body.

4. **Rehmannia (rehmannia glutinosa)**
   This herb acts as a support for the adrenal glands, helpful for people suffering from general debility, and adrenal depletion.
   Note: dose:750-2,250 mg per day up to 4 g per day (tablet or liquid form)

5. **Astragalus (astragalus mambranaceus)**
   An herb used as a combination to support the adrenal glands. This can affect the growth hormones, blood glucose, blood pressure and water balance in the body.
   Note: dose – 2.5-3.4 g daily (benefits after 4-8 weeks)

All these herbs have qualities and used in combination for desired outcomes. Licorine gives immediate remedy with fast and evident results. Ashwagandha and Rhodolia support inner strength, libido and endurance and mental clarity. Korean Ginseng has excellent support for adrenal and thyroid function. Rehmannia is effective for reduction of adrenal fatigue from hypothyroid and hyperthyroid conditions. Astragalus is effective for patients who are tired and struggle during menstrual period in women.

The benefits show patients not feeling tired and not crying for any reason; others improve in energy, lessen or eradicate depression, eliminate hopelessness, think clearly and solve complex decisions on your own. Cortisol secretion becomes normalized and often improves sleep patterns as a result of the normal decrease of cortisol at bedtime.

A lot of factors lead to stress over time so it cannot be resolved overnight, patients need to keep in mind that these herbal therapies usually gauge results after 30-60 days. For chronic exhaustion and helplessness you may take herbal therapies for 30 days more but will need to continue for another 30 days before they start to feel effects.

Chapter 8
How To Combat Adrenal Fatigue Using Natural Method

An individual may fix their adrenal problem temporary by making changes in their lifestyle, but if you can't release all negative emotions that dominate stress it will be useless. We need balance in our body. We cannot perform efficiently if one of the areas in our body is malfunctioning. Adrenal fatigue is cured, you just have to be patient even though it may be long for the recovery to take place.

✓**Removal of stressors**

This is the primary thing that you need to do. This may be emotional coming from marital, finances, family, work and relationships. This needs to be corrected.
Laugh or smile!

✓**Sleep**

Sleep at least 7-8 hours a day for you adrenal glands to repair and recover from wear and tear. Our bodies won't regenerate and function very well to manage stress the
next day if you are deprived from sleep. Listen to soft music to enhance and respond to sleep, have warm baths or read melodramatic stories. You should rest in a dark room to maximize melatonin production.

✓Avoid coffee and carbonated drinks

These are stimulants that interrupt sleep patterns. It is better to drink herbal tea or milk instead.

✓Avoid TV, radio and computers

Some people cannot sleep if they see any form of light. If you are finished watching or using your computer, turn it off and go directly to bed, don't sleep in a chair or so because more or less your sleep will be disrupted.

✓Exercise

The rule of thumb is to stop if tired.

This is a good stress moderator. It normalizes the levels of hormones. It allows the release of carbon dioxide and inhales to expand for oxygen to circulate in the body.

People with adrenal fatigue should not exercise vigorously because it will likely damage the adrenal glands.

- Aerobics such as brisk walking, stair climbing, swimming and treadmill
- Anaerobic, such as weight lifting, pushups, sit ups
- Flexibility such as pilates, stretching, yoga and tai chi
- Meditation
- Deep breathing exercises - instead of jumping out of your seat during traffic jams or other stressful situations, start breathing deeply because according to research it shows that even a few minutes of deep breathing can have an impact on the adrenal glands by reducing the stress hormones they secrete.

✓Nutrition

1. Vitamin C: 500-3000mg. it works better if combined with sodium ascorbate. Consuming foods high in vitamin C, such as oranges and other citrus fruits reduces stress and boost the immune system. Intake of this vitamin can help lower the levels of cortisol, a stress hormone, and blood pressure during high-anxiety situations.

2. Vitamin E: 400-800 IU daily

3. Vitamin B5: 900-1500 mg

4. Vitamin D: 1000-5000 IU, a good nutrient to support hormonal synthesis

5. **Additional nutrients:**
   - 10,000 to 25,000 I.U of beta-carotene
   - selenium (100-200 mcg)
   - magnesium (200-800 mg)
   - lysine (1-2 gm), proline (500mg – 1gm)
   - glutamine (1-5 gm), DHEA 15-50 mg
   - pregnenolone 25-50 mg
   - Ribose and co-factors 2,000-10,000 mg
   - CoQ 300-1,000 mg
   - Type 1 and Type 3 collagen

6. **Steroids**: Matural hydrocortisone or cortisone acetate in doses of 2.5 to 5 mg two to four times a day can be a safe and effective way to replenish depleted adrenals for a short time in very severe case when properly supervised.

7. Complex Carbohydrates: whole grains, fruits, and vegetables, can induce the brain to increase serotonin production and stabilizing blood pressure as a way to reduce stress.

8. Magnesium: Obtaining an adequate amount of magnesium is essential in avoiding headaches and fatigue. Oral magnesium can also successfully relieve premenstrual mood changes. Additionally, increased magnesium intake has been found to improve sleep quality in older adults. Healthy sources of magnesium include spinach or other leafy greens, salmon, and soybeans.

9. Omega-3 Fatty Acids: Fatty fish (such as salmon and tuna) and nuts and seeds (such as flaxseeds, pistachios, walnuts, and almonds) are rich in omega-3 fatty acids, which have been shown to reduce surges of stress hormones and also confer protection against heart disease, depression, and premenstrual syndrome.

10. Because most individuals with adrenal fatigue have compromised digestion, it is important that they can digest food and supplement intake properly and have gastric flora balance.

You may want to include the following in your daily diet to assist in adrenal restoration:
- Probiotics - 2 to 3 times per day
- Digestive enzymes that are taken-in with every meals
- Eating raw fermented vegetables – daily

1.Eat plentiful amounts of fresh fruits and vegetables.

2.Try to have a small garden in your backyard. Plant crops that are not sprayed with pesticides so that increased intake of these nutrients will combat stress which depletes these nutrients.

Chapter 9
A Practical Eating Plan To Help Prevent And Combat Adrenal Fatigue

Between 6am and 8am studies shows that cortisol levels peak and you may not have the urgency to eat. A lot of people, including myself, don't eat breakfast because "I am not hungry". However, skipping meals, especially breakfast is not a good idea because it is the most important meal of the day.

Once the body senses that you are low in sugar, the neurotransmitters instruct the adrenals to secrete cortisol to activate gluconeogenesis and increase the blood glucose level which allows the body to function normally. So, have a healthy breakfast soon after waking, but do not eat later than 10 a.m.

From 11:00 am to 11:30am, is the best time for lunch to be served. To sustain our bodies from alterations in the normal cortisol levels which occur between 3:00-4:00pm, it is advisable to have a snack between 2:00-3:00pm.

Supper should be served around 5:00-6:00 pm. If necessary, meals should be in small proportions and low in sugar to avoid an increase in the blood sugar. Symptoms such as anxiety and night sweats are seen and the body then sends a signal to the adrenals for more cortisol to normalize the blood sugar level. If this happens year after year, this will cause an excessive burden to the adrenal glands.

Chapter 10
Natural Ways To Relieve Stress

It's impractical to just walk away from problems, so rather face them not with fear but with confidence. Our world is fast paced, if a person stops it will be hard to recoup and get back on track again. Stress drains everything and if you let yourself be affected, you will see it through physical, emotional and/or mental distress. Taking stress medications are not always a good thing because stress can be prevented and cured by how a person manages everything in life.

These are the natural ways to help reduce our stress levels.

1. Walking
Fresh air does so many things to our senses and well-being. Walking at least 30 minutes a day will increase your mental sharpness.

2. Write
Having your own journal is therapeutic. It's a way people express their thoughts and feelings giving the mind focus which becomes a good tool for problem solving.

3. Exercise
There are a lot of exercises to choose from. They can range from engaging in moderate to the high level of exercise. Workouts set you away from thinking about your problems, becoming calm and relaxing the body from stressful situations. During exercise, hormones

are released and bring an individual to balance. It is also proven that when exercising, a person will sleep better and have a stronger immune system.

4.Deep breathing

Releasing the stored carbon dioxide is very important as well as oxygen coming into our body to circulate and provide us a greater level of equilibrium. Deep breathing gives us a sense of inner peace and tranquility and frees us from the negativity of stressors and environment. The best part is that you can do this anytime, no specific steps to follow but only takes a few minutes of your time to be still, enjoy the quietness and clear your mind of all life's distractions.

5. Laughter

"Laughter is the best medicine" whoever said this, is definitely right. You always feel relieved when you have a good laugh; you feel more light-hearted and have a more positive outlook.

6.Eating well

I often hear people say "you are what you eat" and yes I can say that is true. There is lot of refined food which makes us more inclined to grab it in the grocery due to our hectic lives. Planning a home cooked meal and setting a time maybe around 30 minutes to treat our body and have the nutrients that it needs to feel energized and function effectively throughout the day.

7. Listen to music

Music keeps you moving. You can listen to any music that suits your needs, this will help you relax and meditate.

8. Tea

There are a lot of teas available that you can choose from. This brings relaxation and calmness to your life. These are antioxidant, which help you get free radicals rather than coffee. Caffeine is also present in tea, so it is also recommended that you follow the proper level directions in how often you consume it. Even if the world is moving at a fast pace, take the time to slow down, breathe and take it one day at a time.

Conclusion:

As we live and face each day, we are disturbed with so many trials and challenges that we need to solve in order to survive. It is a relief that we have our adrenal glands that help us cope, survive our ordeals in life and function efficiently all throughout our body. We may not feel it every day, but it appears and comes in disguise that we are not even aware of. This may be a combination of physical, emotional, psychological, environmental, perceived and infectious because our adrenal glands work together within our body and our mind to respond in battling off stressors that may come.

We are not like the people in fictional stories such as superwoman or supermen that seem to be perfect with no flaws. We are human beings and we are what we make of our body. From both my personal and professional experience, I understand and appreciate the impact when my adrenal glands and body are not working in unanimity. Every now and then we need to look beyond conventional medicine towards alternative forms for therapy to achieve and to live a healthy lifestyle at an optimum level. Love yourself, your body and everything else will follow.

www.ingramcontent.com/pod-product-compliance
Lightning Source LLC
Chambersburg PA
CBHW070236290526
45789CB00004B/1649

* 9 781502 390691 *